WALL PILATES

WORKOUTS BIBLE

FOR WOMEN

THE COMPLETE 30-DAY BODY SCULPTING CHALLENGE TO TONE YOUR GLUTES, ABS & BACK

COLOR EDITION - 2023

Copyright Notice:

© [2023] [Christian Walton]. All rights reserved.

No part of this publication may be reproduced, distributed, or transmitted in any form or by any means, including photocopying, recording, or other electronic or mechanical methods, without the prior written permission of the publisher, except in the case of brief quotations embodied in reviews and certain other noncommercial uses permitted by copyright law.

Disclaimer:

This book is provided for informational purposes only and is not intended to replace professional medical advice, diagnosis, or treatment. Consult with a qualified healthcare provider before beginning any new exercise program, especially if you have any pre-existing health conditions or concerns. The author and publisher disclaim any liability or loss in connection with the exercises, opinions, or information expressed in this book. Any application of the material provided is at the reader's discretion and sole responsibility.

CONTENTS

INTRODUCTION 8

FULL BODY 10

CARDIO 40

CORE 56

30-Day Body Sculpting Challenge 72

Tracking the 30-Day Challenge 103

PDF BONUS 104

FULL BODY – PAGE 10

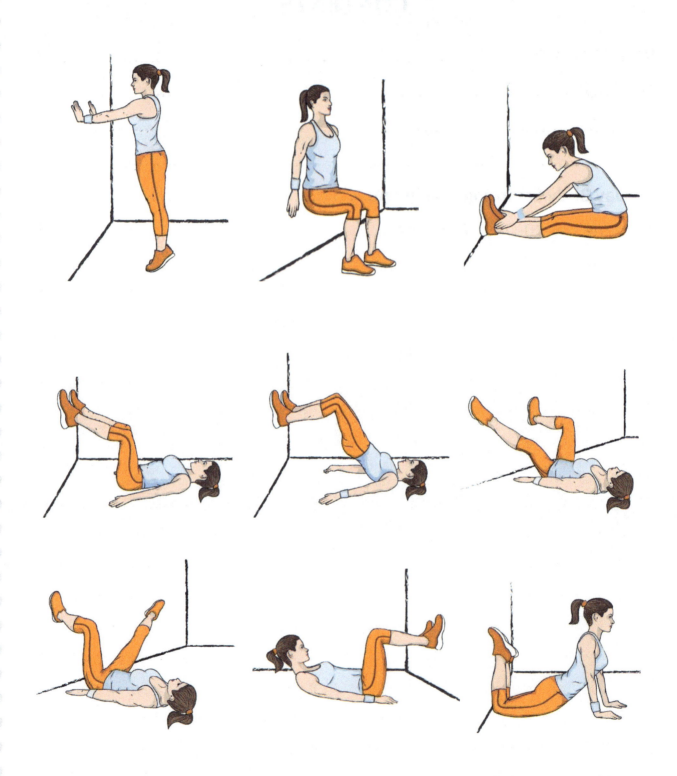

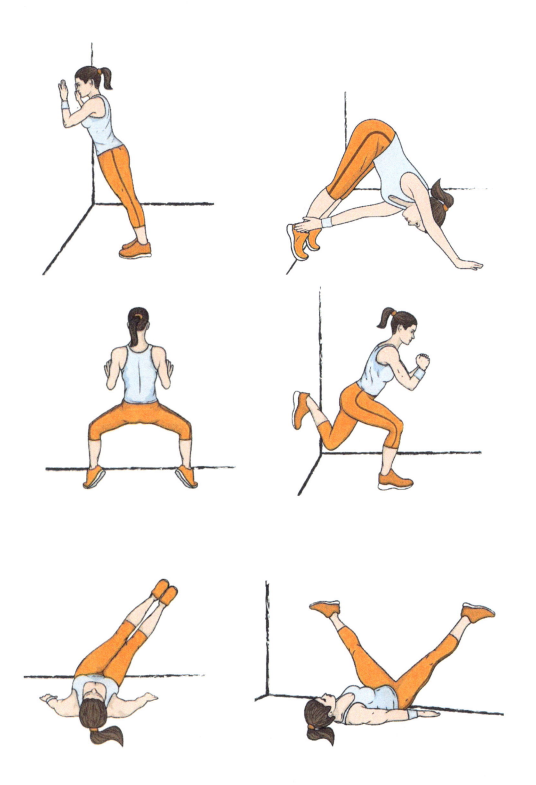

CARDIO – PAGE 40

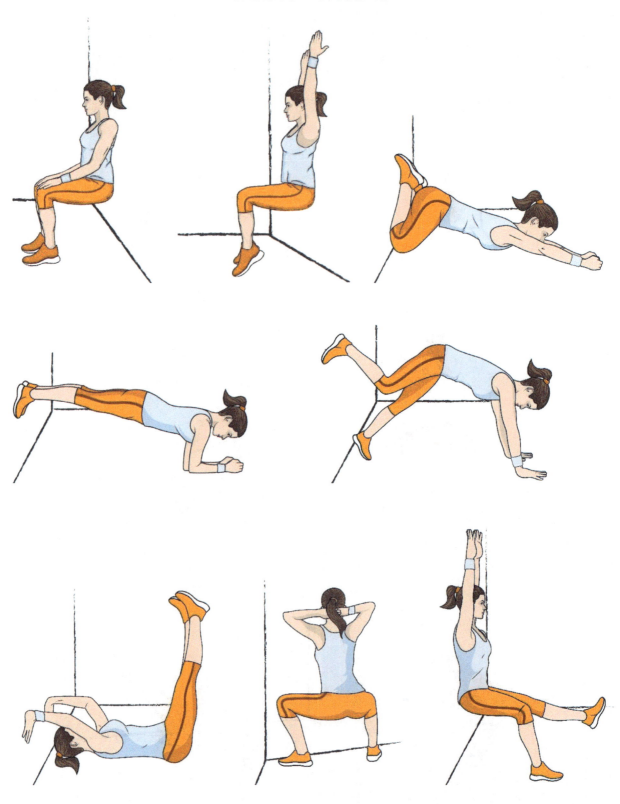

CORE – PAGE 56

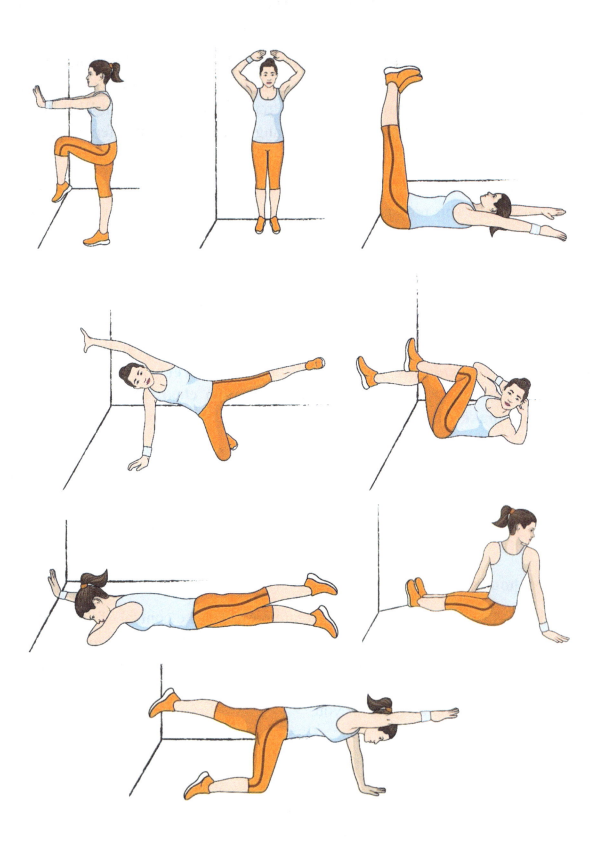

INTRODUCTION

Welcome to "Wall Pilates Workouts Bible for Women: The Complete 30-Day Body Sculpting Challenge". As a personal fitness trainer with over a decade of experience in the industry, I have seen fitness trends come and go. But Wall Pilates is not just another fleeting trend; it's a game-changing practice that offers unparalleled benefits for women of all ages and fitness levels.

Wall Pilates is a fusion of classical Pilates principles with the support and challenge of a wall. This unique combination allows greater stability while providing a way to deepen stretches, engage muscles more fully, and bring a new dimension to traditional Pilates routines. Whether you are a seasoned Pilates enthusiast or new to the world of fitness, the benefits of Wall Pilates can transform your daily life.

What's Inside?

This 30-Day challenge is designed to engage your body, sculpt your glutes, abs, and back, and enhance your overall flexibility, strength, and balance. The routines are crafted to be simple yet effective, with clear, illustrated full-body exercises that make following along a breeze.

The book offers a *detailed day-by-day guide* with fresh, engaging routines to keep you motivated and challenged to work on your body and health. Through persistence and dedication, you will see tangible results.

The transformation is not just physical but mental as well.

For whom is this book?

This book is crafted for women who are ready to take control of their fitness in an entirely new way. It's for those who crave something more than just another routine, something that speaks to both the body and soul. Whether you're looking to kickstart your fitness journey, break through a plateau, or add a fresh twist to your existing regimen, this 30-day challenge is for you.

And the best part is:

You can see amazing results just by doing Pilates exercises for 10 to 15 minutes a day!

BENEFITS OF DOING 30-DAY WALL PILATES FOR YOUR BODY:

1. **Improved posture**
2. **Toned glutes, abs and back**
3. **Boost in energy level**
4. **Reduction of stress level**
5. **Slimmer waist**
6. **Improved flexibility, strength, and balance**
7. **And much more…**

Embrace the Challenge

I invite you to embark on this transformative journey with me.

With commitment, courage, and the guidance laid out in these pages, you'll forge a stronger, more confident, and balanced version of yourself.

Your ultimate body sculpting challenge awaits.

Let's embrace it together and shape your dream body.

Welcome to the world of Wall Pilates.

FULL BODY

WALL CALF RAISES

How to do it:

1. Stand facing the wall and place your palms against the wall to create support.
2. Raise your heels as high as you can, tensing all the muscles in your legs.
3. Lower your heels.
4. Repeat.

Note: it is important to keep your knees straight during the entire exercise.

The benefits of the exercise: the exercise improves posture, strengthens the ankle joint and foot, and improves the technique of performing other exercises.

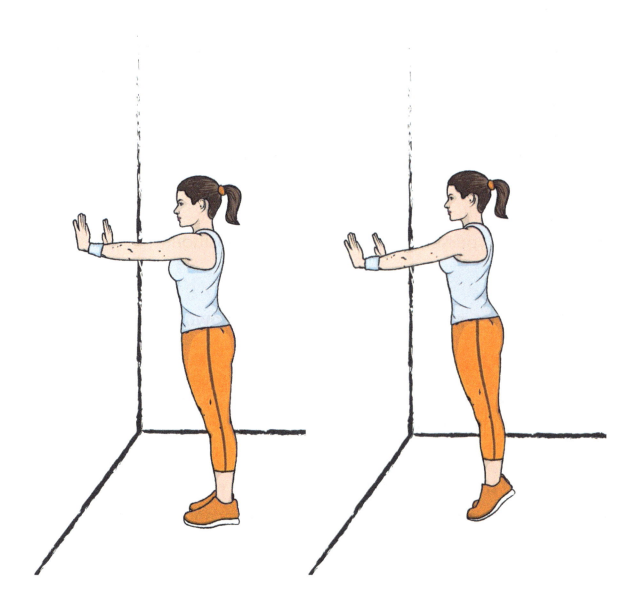

WALL SIT WITH LEG EXTENSION

How to do it:

1. Stand with your back to the wall, a short step away, with your feet shoulder-width apart, and a 90° angle should form at the knees (see illustration).
2. Press your back and head against the wall. Tighten your belly.
3. Place your palms against the wall and slowly, lift upwards without taking your feet off the floor so that your legs are completely straight (see illustration).
4. Then lower yourself down to the starting position.

Exhale as you go up and inhale as you go down.

Note: This exercise is best done in clothing with sleeves, as it will make it easier to slide along the wall.

The benefits of the exercise: strengthening and working out the muscles of the legs and buttocks; improving body stability and balance.

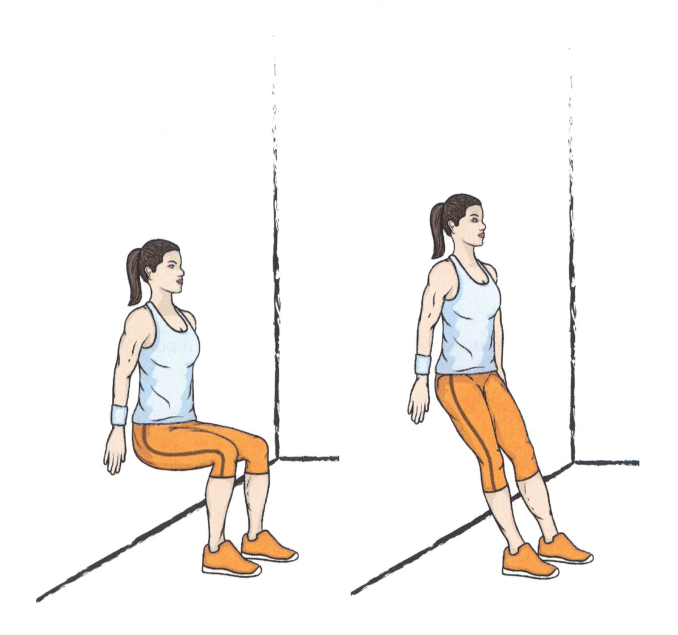

TILT THE BODY FORWARD

How to do it:

1. Sit up straight, straighten your legs, and press your feet against the wall.
2. Straighten your back and start inhaling, stretching upward.
3. As you exhale, gently bend down to your feet, try to stretch your arms and back well, and feel your legs, especially the back of them, as you bend down.

Note: during this exercise, you should firmly feel the support of your feet against the wall.

The benefits of the exercise: this exercise works the abdominal muscles (abs) and back, as well as the gluteal muscles and the back of the thigh.

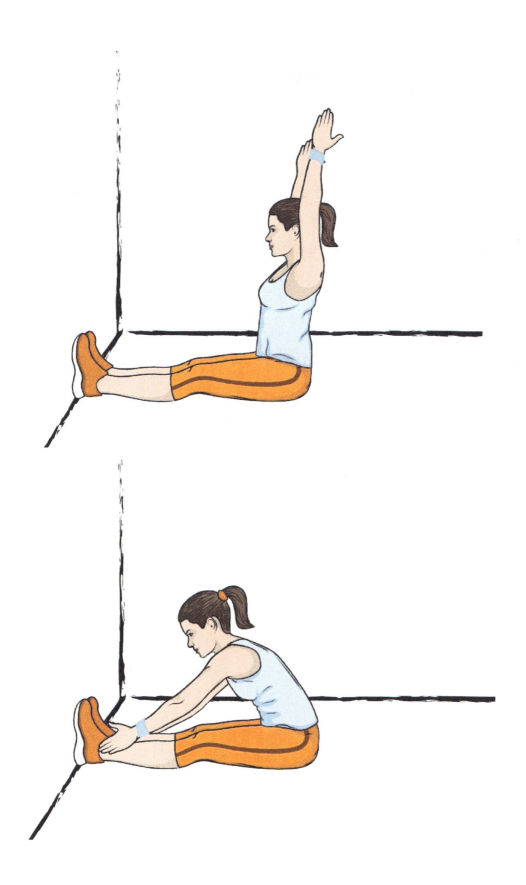

15

WALL BRIDGE

How to do it:

1. Lie on your back, move a little closer to the wall, and place your feet on the wall so that your knees form an angle of approximately 90°.
2. Begin to perform gentle and smooth pelvic lifts upward.
3. Exhale when lifting the pelvis and inhale when lowering it.

Note: when we lift the pelvis up, we rest our heels well against the wall.

The benefits of the exercise: the biceps of the thighs (the muscles of the back of the leg) and back muscles are worked out; the exercise improves the support and stability of the pelvis and spine.

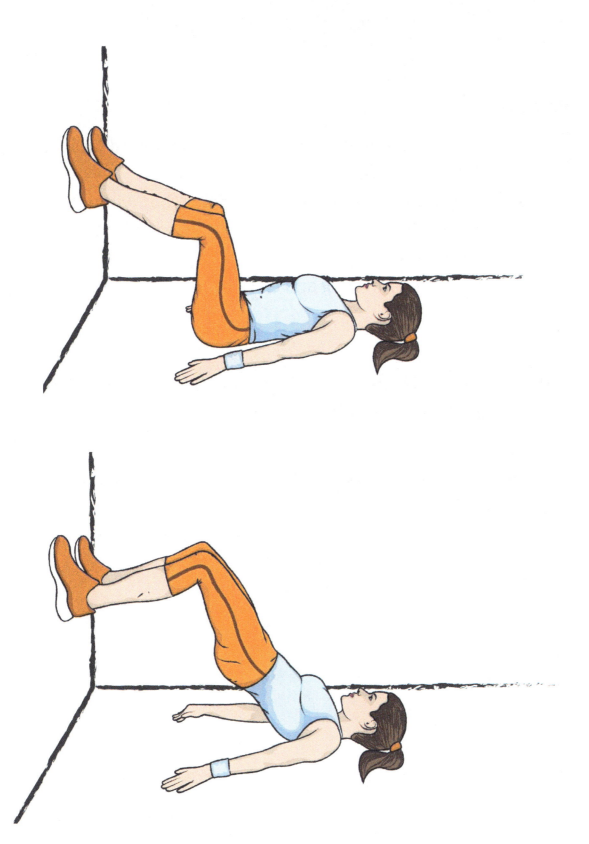

SMALL PELVIC LIFTS

How to do it:

1. Stay in the same position with the pelvis raised (as in the previous exercise). See illustrations.
2. Start pulsing your pelvis up and down, but without lowering it to the floor. The amplitude should not be too big for safety. Listen to the sensations in your body.
3. Inhale when lowering and exhale when raising the pelvis.

Note: you don't need to do the exercises quickly, because Pilates against the wall is all about feeling the muscles and engaging them deeper.

The benefits of the exercise: strengthening the gluteal muscles, improving balance and endurance.

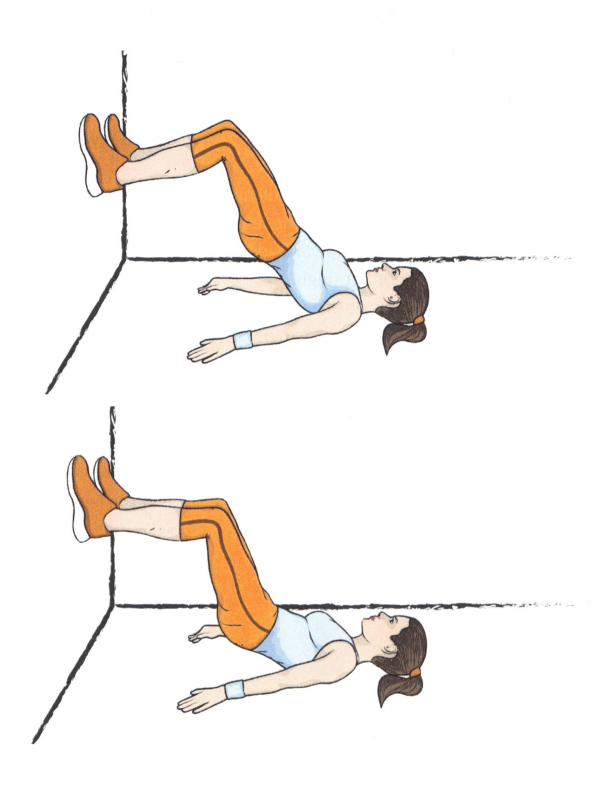

WALL SINGLE LEG STRETCH (Left)

How to do it:

1. Lie on the floor and place your feet on the wall so that your knees are at an angle of approximately 90°.
2. Straighten your left leg upward, pulling with your fingertips, and begin to perform abduction to the left side.
3. Keep your foot extended upward and your muscles tight, trying to feel the inside of your left thigh.
4. Move your leg to the side as far as possible for you.
5. Inhale as you lift your leg and exhale as you move it to the side.

Note: keep your lower back well pressed to the floor and your abs tight.

The benefits of the exercise: stretching the muscles of the hips and legs, which helps to improve flexibility and reduce tension in the legs; working the muscles of the abs and back, as well as the gluteal muscles.

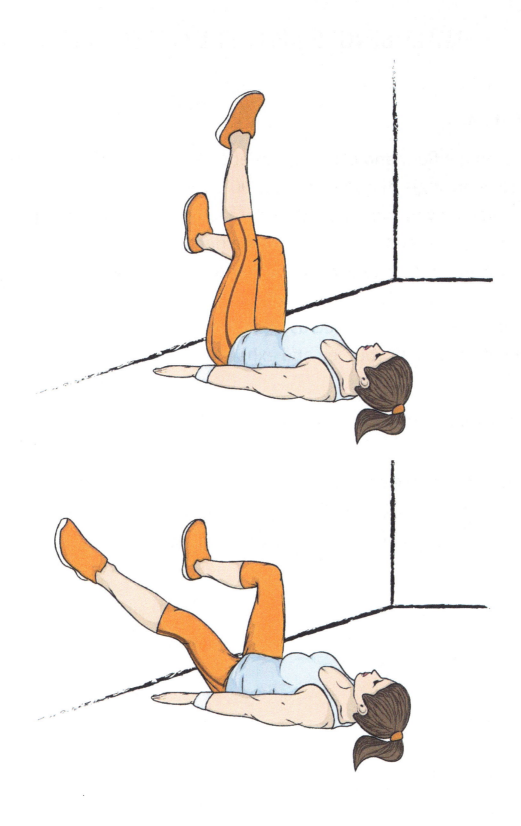

WALL SINGLE LEG STRETCH (Right)

How to do it:

1. Lie on the floor and place your feet on the wall so that your knees are at an angle of approximately 90°.
2. Straighten your right leg upward, reaching out with your fingertips, and begin to abduct your leg to the right side.
3. Keep your foot extended upward and your muscles tight, trying to feel the inside of your left thigh.
4. Move your leg to the side as far as possible.
5. Inhale as you lift your leg and exhale as you move it to the side.

Note: keep your lower back well pressed to the floor and your abs tight.

The benefits of the exercise: stretching the muscles of the hips and legs, which helps to improve flexibility and reduce tension in the legs; works the muscles of the abs and back, as well as the gluteal muscles.

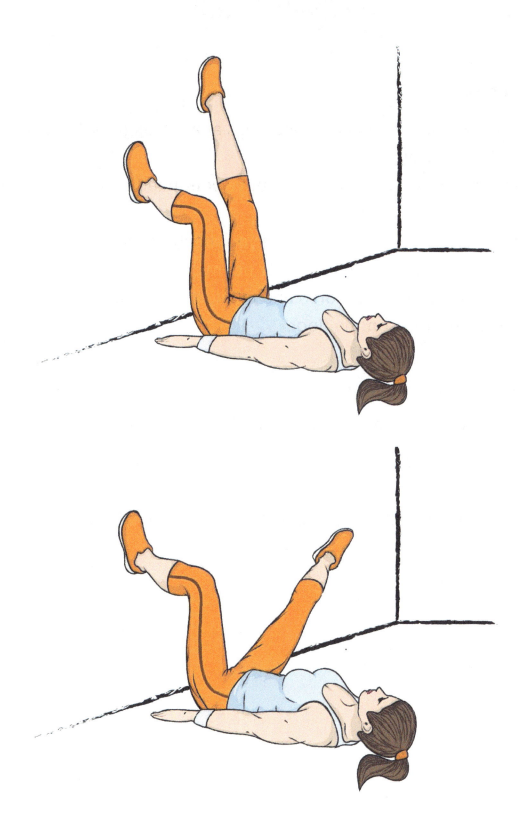

LEGS-UP CRUNCH

How to do it:

1. Lie on your back and place your legs at a 90° angle with your feet against the wall.
2. Stretch your arms behind you above your head with your hands on the floor (see illustrations).
3. Start doing a gentle twist, lifting your head and shoulders while lowering your hands to the floor near your hips.
4. Exhale as you lift your torso and inhale as you lower it to the starting position on the floor.

Note: It is very important that your lower back is well-pressed to the floor throughout the exercise. And to get a little higher on the turn, press your heels hard into the wall.

The benefits of the exercise: strengthening abdominal muscles (abs).

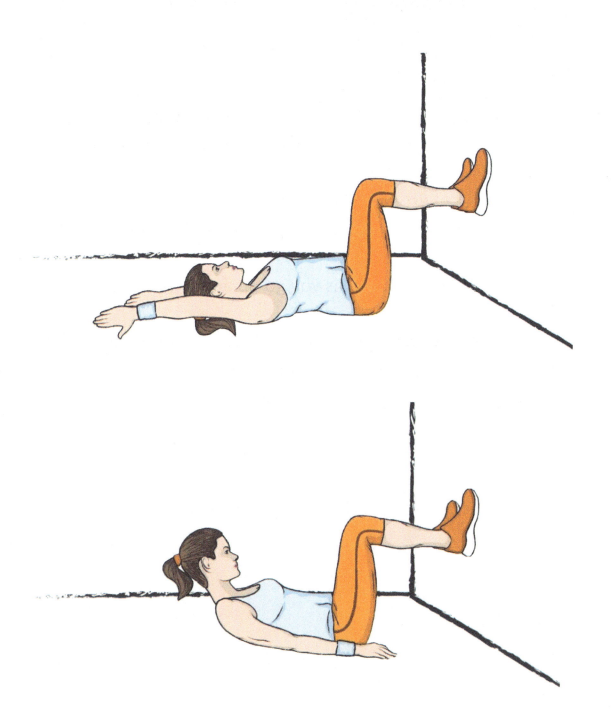

WALL COBRA STRETCH

How to do it:

1. Lie on the mat facing the floor with your chest touching the mat and your knees resting against the wall, your shins pressed against the wall.
2. Arms bent at chest level, palms resting on the floor.
3. From this position, lift your chest and head, helping yourself with your hands.
4. Exhale through your nose as you go up and inhale as you go down.

The benefits of the exercise: improving spinal flexibility, training the muscles of the back and buttocks; improving posture and flexibility of the whole body.

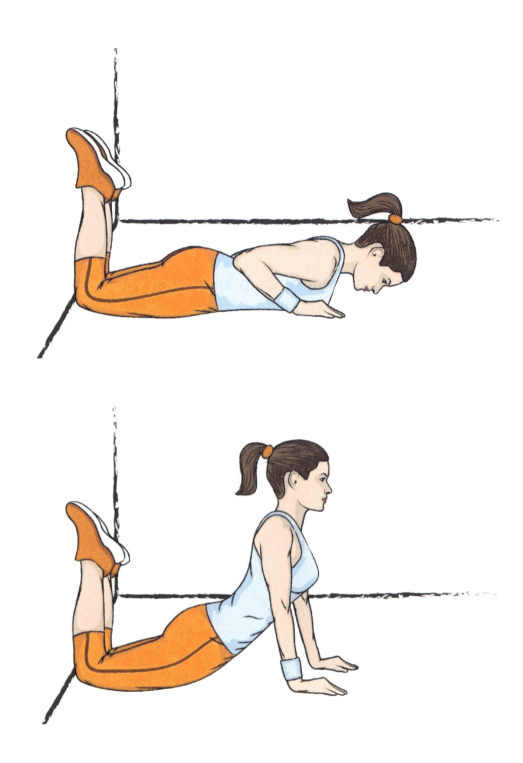

TOE TOUCH CRUNCH

How to do it:

1. Face the mat with your arms straight and your feet against the wall (see illustration).

2. As you exhale, lift your hips up and touch your right ankle with your left hand.

3. While inhaling, return to the starting position.

4. As you exhale, lift your hips up and touch your left ankle with your opposite (right) hand.

5. Then, as you inhale, return to the starting position.

The benefits of the exercise: train the transverse abdominal muscles, arm muscles, and lower abs; strengthen the muscles of the whole body.

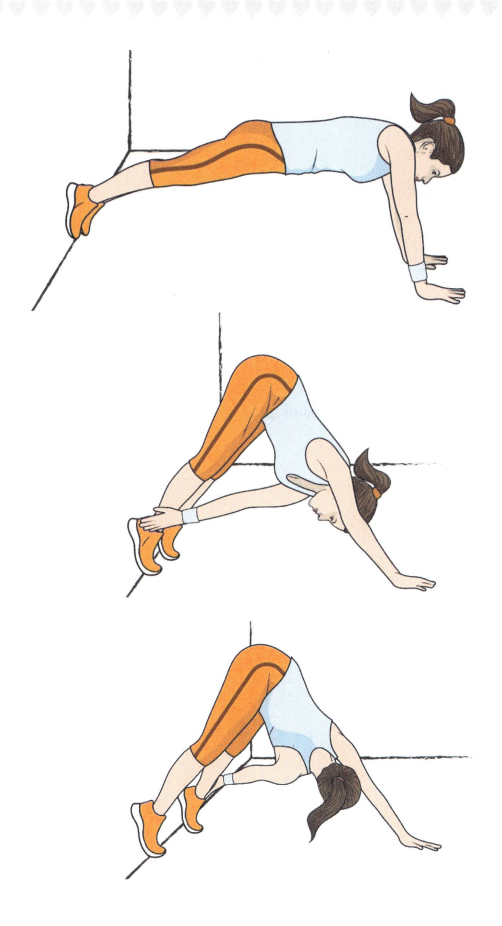

WALL PUSH-UP

How to do it:

1. Stand facing the wall, a short step away.
2. Place your elbows shoulder-width apart on the wall, palms facing up, as shown in the illustration.
3. When pressing your arms against the wall, straighten your elbows so that your arms are in a straight position on the wall. It is important not to lift your heels off the floor.
4. Then slowly return to the starting position with your elbows bent on the wall.
5. Exhale as you push off the wall and inhale as you return to the starting position.

The benefits of the exercise: strengthening the muscles of the chest, shoulder girdle and arms, increasing overall arm strength.

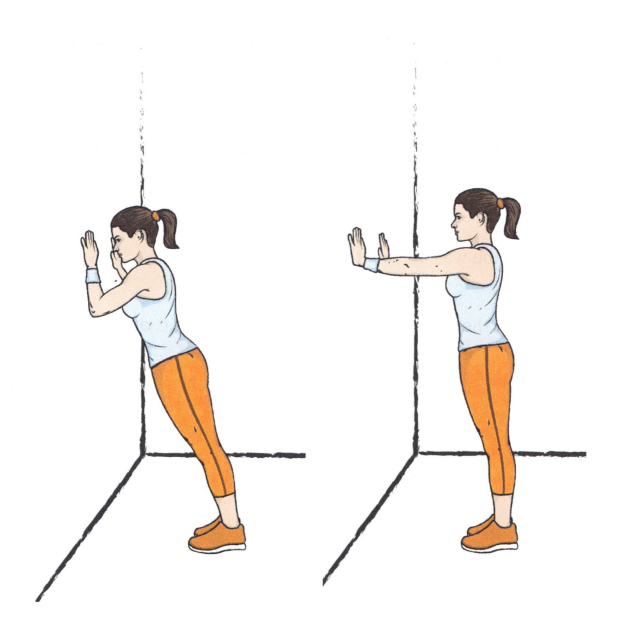

31

LIFTING ON THE TOES

How to do it:

1. Stand facing the wall, a short distance away (short step). Place your hands in front of you, palms facing the wall for support.
2. Bend your knees about 90° and spread your legs apart as much as possible.
3. Inhale - lift your heels off the floor, exhale - lower your heels to the floor.

Note: Lean on the wall only with your hands.

The benefits of the exercise: strengthening the muscles of the thighs and buttocks, the lower body becomes slim and toned.

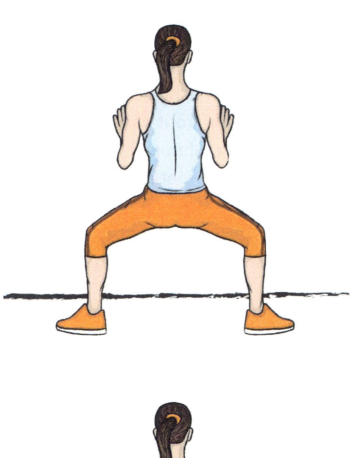
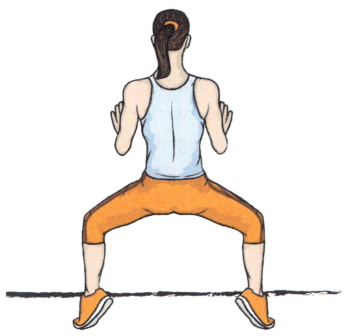

WALL SQUATS ON ONE LEG

How to do it:

1. Stand with your back to the wall at a step distance.
2. Place your left foot on the wall behind you at about hip level.
3. Keep your hands together in front of your chest.
4. Begin to slowly squat down, shifting most of your body weight to your right leg, while your left foot is pressed firmly against the wall to help maintain balance.
5. Straighten your right leg to return to the starting position.
6. Exhale when you squat and inhale when you straighten your knee.

Repeat the exercise for the left leg.

Note: leaning your body forward is normal; the more you lean forward, the more your glutes will work.

The benefits of the exercise: develops leg muscles, as well as strengthens the abs and sense of balance; the exercise increases endurance and strength; trains the quadriceps and gluteus maximus muscles.

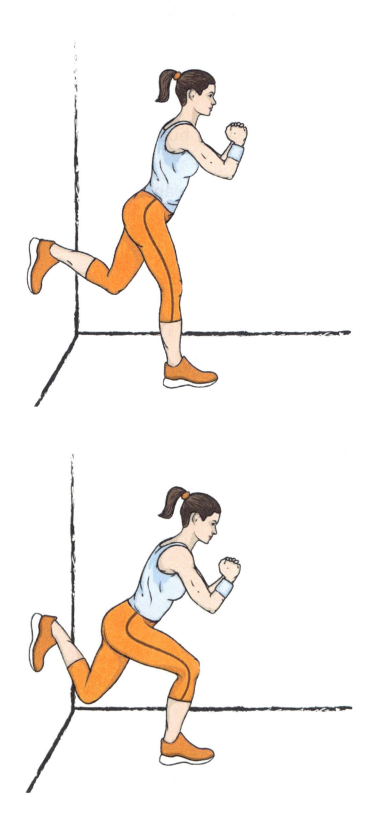

WALL LEG LIFTS

How to do it:

1. Lie back on the mat with your buttocks fully against the wall. Keep your legs straight up.
2. Arms straight on the floor, wide apart, palms down, for a sense of support.
3. Now move both legs together to the right and then to the left, keeping your hands on the floor.
4. Breathe steadily and deeply throughout the exercise. Exhale as you swing your legs to the sides and inhale as you move your legs back to the starting position (legs up).

The benefits of the exercise: improves blood circulation, flexibility of the lumbar spine, and trains the lower abdominal muscles.

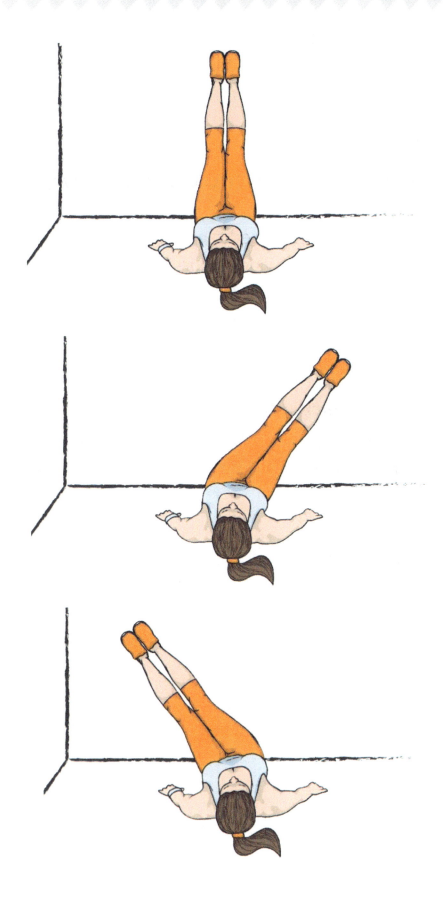

WALL SCISSOR

How to do it:

1. Lie back on the mat (floor) with your buttocks fully against the wall (see the illustration).
2. The legs are raised up, pressed together.
3. Now spread your legs as wide as possible and move your feet apart.
4. Hold this position for 5 seconds.
5. Put your legs together, relaxing your muscles (starting position).

The benefits of the exercise: toning of the thigh muscles and adductor muscles; strengthening of the pelvic muscles, activation of blood flow; training of the press and inner thigh.

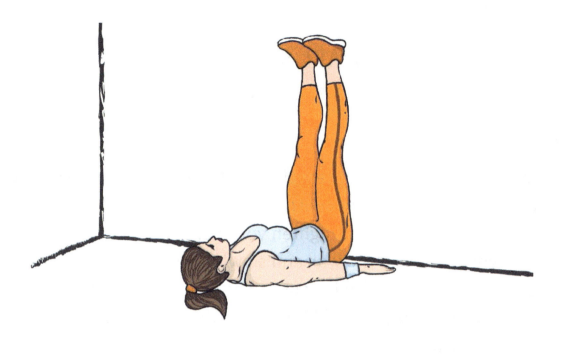

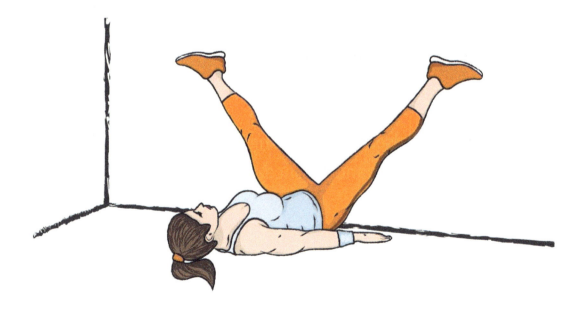

CARDIO

WALL SQUATS

How to do it:

1. Stand with your back to the wall, at a distance of a small step, with your feet shoulder-width apart.
2. Lean against the wall and tighten your belly.
3. Place your palms on the wall and slowly slide down the wall as if you were sitting on a chair. Your thighs should be parallel to the floor and your knees should form a 90° angle. Press your back and head well against the wall.
4. Breathe deeply: inhale through your nose and exhale through your mouth. You will feel all the muscles in your body tense up.
5. Hold the pose for 10-15 seconds, then slowly return to a straight leg position, relaxing your muscles.

The benefits of the exercise: strengthening gluteal muscles and quadriceps, improving strength, stability and balance.

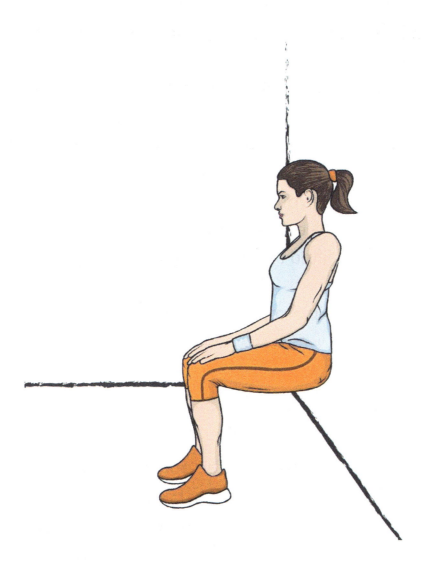

WALL SIT HEEL RAISE

How to do it:

1. Stand with your back to the wall, one small step apart, feet shoulder-width apart.
2. Place your palms on the wall and, with your back and head firmly against the wall, slowly lower yourself down as if you were sitting in a chair. Thighs should be parallel to the floor and knees at a 90° angle.
3. Lift your heels, shifting your weight to the front of your feet, while raising your arms. Inhale during this movement.
4. When the heels are lifted as high as possible, you can take a short exhale.
5. Then slowly lower your arms and heels to the floor while exhaling (starting position).

The benefits of the exercise: effective for strengthening leg muscles and developing body stability, helps improve balance and coordination. It is especially useful for people who spend a lot of time at a desk.

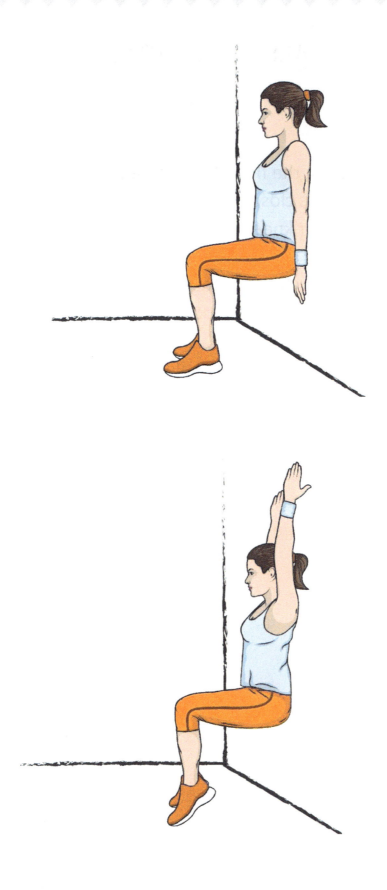

WALL CAT STRETCH

How to do it:

1. Lie on the mat facing the floor, leaning on your elbows, bent at a 90° angle, with your arms closed in front of you.
2. You need to lean your knees against the wall and press your shins against the wall.
3. From this position, try to push back with your arms so that your arms are straight, and your buttocks touch your heels.
4. Return to the starting position.
5. Exhale as you raise your pelvis, inhale as you lower yourself to your elbows.

The benefits of the exercise: the exercise is aimed at stretching and toning the muscles of the back, upper, middle, and lower parts; improving flexibility, increasing the range of motion; relieving tension in the shoulders and neck.

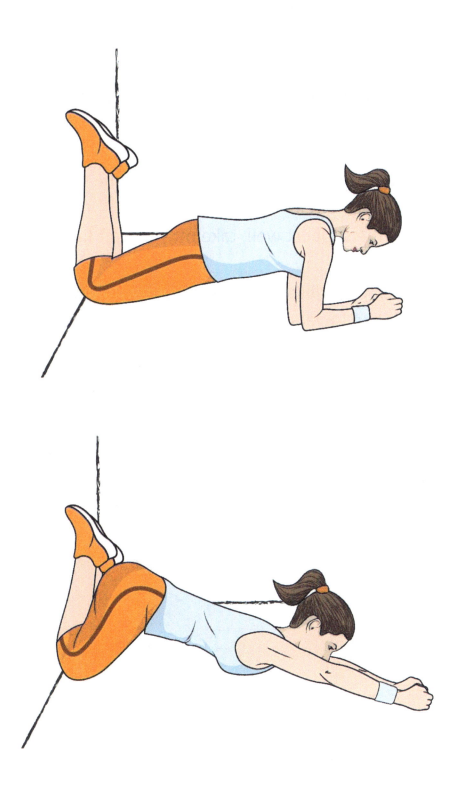

WALL PLANK

How to do it:

1. Get down on your elbows and knees. The angles should be 90° (see the illustration).
2. Now you should straighten your right leg and press it well against the wall so that you can lift your other leg off the ground and press it against the wall as well.
3. Once you feel the support well, take off your left leg and put it against the wall.
4. In this position, you will have to tense your whole body, hold for 3 seconds, and then lower one leg and then the other.

The benefits of the exercise: strengthening of the abdominal muscles and core muscles, in particular, the rectus and transverse abdominis; the exercise activates the deltoid and triceps muscles; maintains good posture and increases strength.

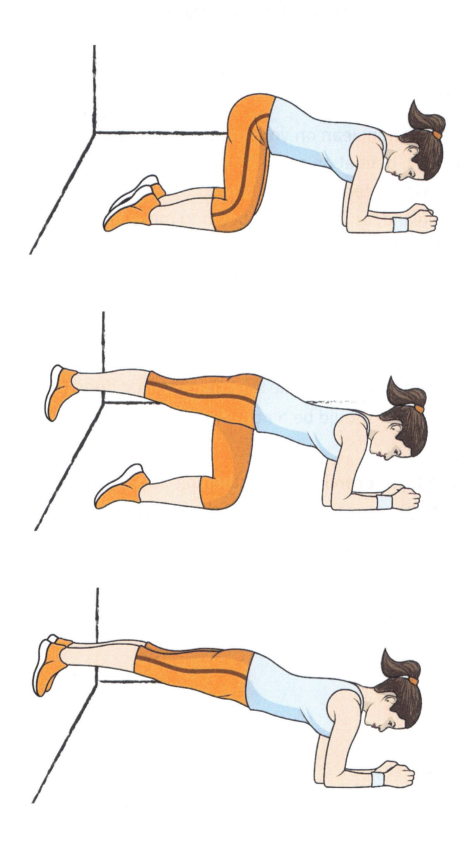

47

CLIMB A MOUNTAIN

How to do it:

1. Starting position: lean on your palms, arms straight, knees shoulder-width apart, bent at an angle of approximately 90°, and the abdomen is tightened (see illustration 1).
2. Breathe in and, as you exhale, begin to move up the wall (see illustration 2).
3. Hold this position for 3-4 seconds (see illustration 3).
4. Return to the starting position for 3-4 seconds.

Note: It is very important to make sure that the mat does not slide forward when you step up; it should be a non-slip surface.

The benefits of the exercise: strengthening and toning the whole body, especially strengthening the muscles of the arms and shoulders, improving posture.

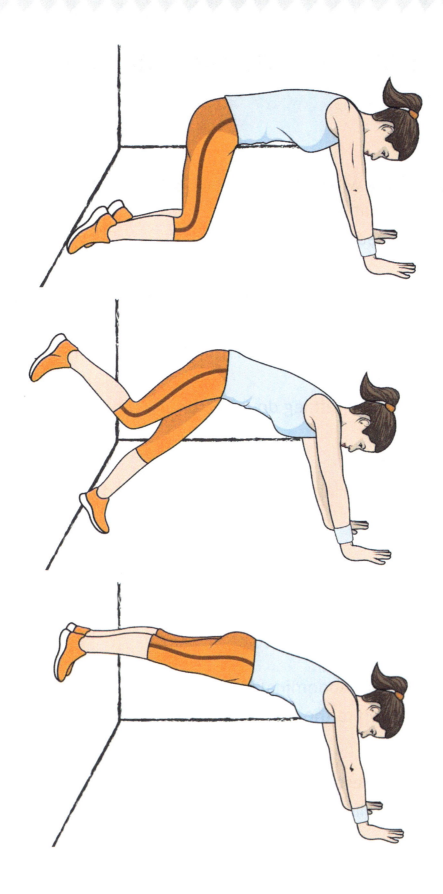

49

LEG LIFT WITH WALL SUPPORT

How to do it:

1. Lie on your back with your palms firmly against the wall behind your head (see illustration).
2. Legs straightened, raised up.

    Step 1: Tighten your abdominal muscles and smoothly, without jerking, lower your right leg down without touching the floor, parallel to the mat, and then lift it up to the starting position.

    Step 2: Lower your left leg down, also without touching the floor, and lift it up.

    Step 3: Lower both legs parallel to the floor and lift to the starting position.

3. Exhale when you lower your legs down, inhale when you raise your legs up.

Note: do not relax your abdominal muscles. Watch where the lower back is, it should be pressed to the floor, this is necessary to maintain its safety.

The benefits of the exercise: all the muscles of the lower abdomen work, improving tone and relief; thigh muscles are strengthened, and endurance increases.

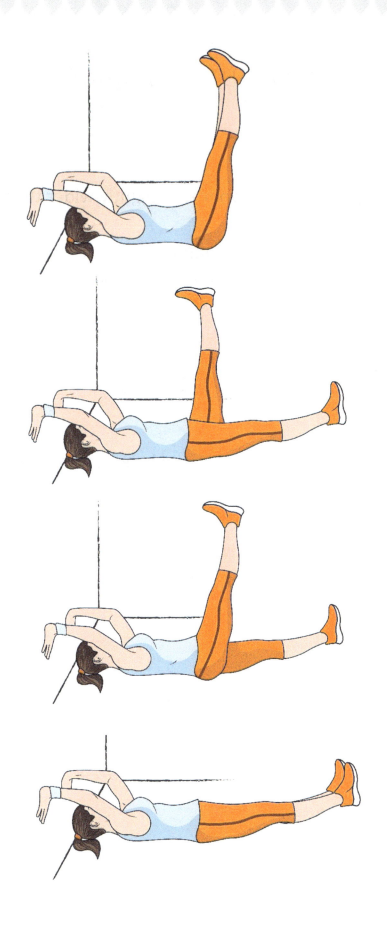

FORWARD WALL SQUATS

How to do it:

1. Stand facing the wall with your feet slightly wider than your shoulders.
2. Stand shoulder-width apart, with your toes resting on the wall and your feet spread apart. Clasp your hands behind your head.
3. Start squatting at a slow pace, going as low as possible.
4. Keep your knees, chest, and face as close to the wall as possible throughout the exercise.
5. Exhale as you squat and inhale as you rise.

Note: the more you spread your feet and knees apart, the more your inner thigh will work.

The benefits of the exercise: activate the gluteal and thigh muscles; increases strength and endurance; strengthens and tone the muscles of the legs and back.

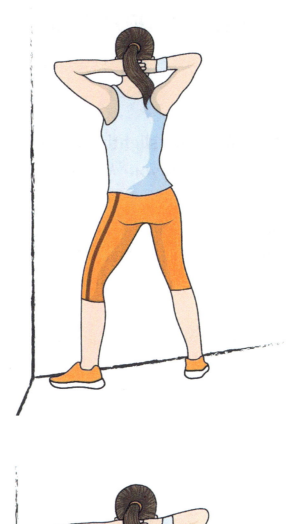
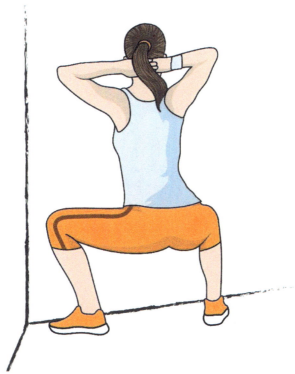

ONE-LEGGED WALL SIT

How to do it:

1. Lean against the wall, knees slightly bent and arms down.
2. Raise your arms and extend your *left leg*.
3. Hold this position for 10 seconds (deep and even inhalation and exhalation of air).
4. Then lower your arms and left leg and pause for 5 seconds.
5. Raise your arms, then straighten your *right leg* and hold for 10 seconds.
6. Then lower your arms and right leg and pause for 5 seconds.

The benefits of the exercise: strengthens and tones the buttocks, quadriceps biceps, works the adductor/abductor muscles of the thighs (inner thigh), calves, and abs.

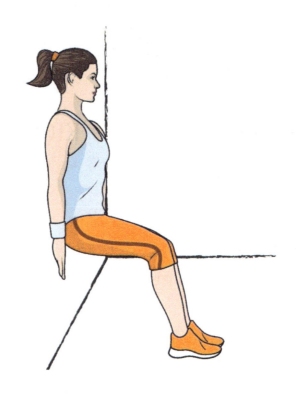

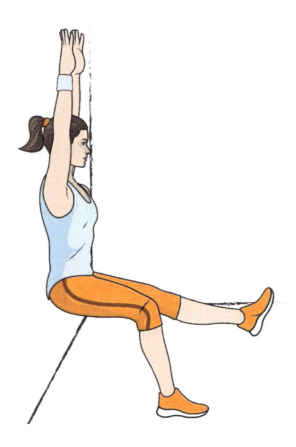

CORE

WALL LEG RAISE + KICK BACK

How to do it:

1. Stand facing the wall, arms straightened in front of you, palms against the wall. Keep your feet shoulder-width apart (see the illustration).
2. As you inhale, lift your *left leg* and extend your knee in front of you as high as possible while standing on your right toes.
3. As you exhale, lower your left leg and lean back, squeezing your buttocks and abs; lower the heel of your right foot to the floor.
4. Do this exercise with your *right leg*.

Note: It is important to perform this exercise slowly, inhaling deeply through the nose and exhaling through the mouth.
Remember to control your back - a natural bend in the lower back is allowed, but no more.

The benefits of the exercise: the muscles of the thighs, buttocks, and lower legs are actively worked and toned, which helps to develop strength and endurance and improve coordination and balance.

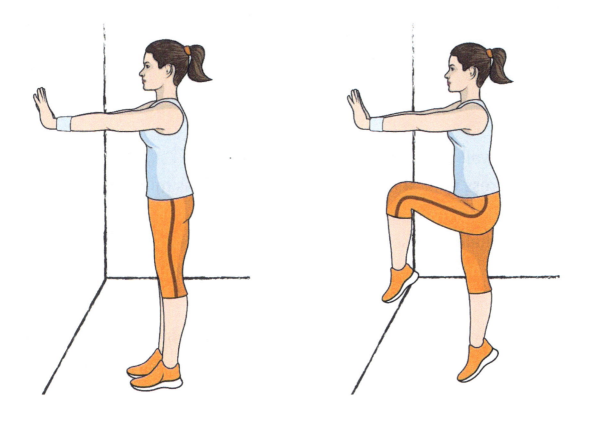

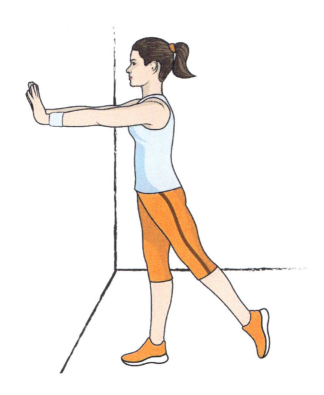

57

WALL ANGELS

How to do it:

1. Go to a wall and lean your back against it.
2. Try to press your shoulders against the wall as much as possible.
3. Raise your arms and press them against the wall (see illustrations).
4. While inhaling, raise your arms up, joining them above your head.
5. As you exhale, lower your arms down to the starting position.

Note: try not to take your hands off the wall (*they should slide along the wall*). Feel your back, arms, and shoulders, also tensing your abs.

The benefits of the exercise: improves posture and engages the deep back muscles; relieves tension in the back.

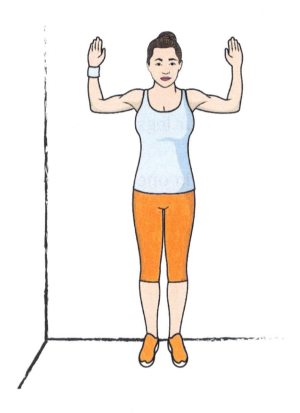

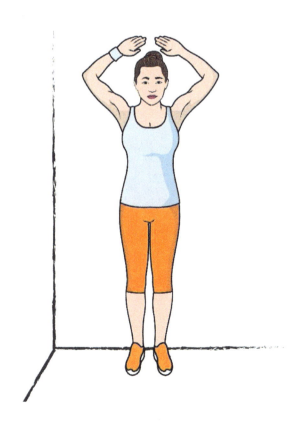

SEATED TRUNK ROTATION

How to do it:

1. Sit up straight, straighten your legs and back with your feet against the wall.
2. Start turning your torso first in one direction and then in the other, extending your straight arm as far as possible.
3. Exhale as you turn to the right or left, touching the floor with your hands.
4. Inhale in the middle position - when you are facing the wall.

The benefits of the exercise: the exercise activates the muscles of the face and back, improves spinal flexibility; improves blood circulation in the muscles and joints.

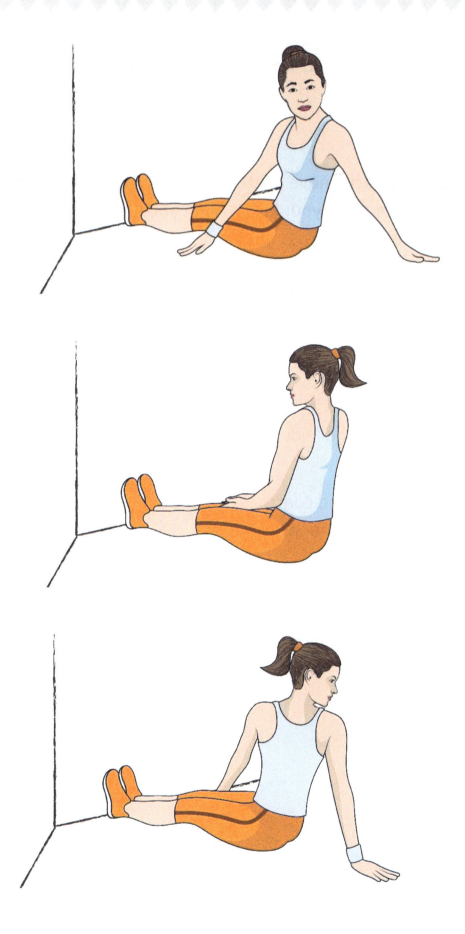

WALL BICYCLE CRUNCHES

How to do it:

1. Lie on your back, move a little closer to the wall, and place your feet on the wall so that your knees form about a 90° angle (see illustration).
2. Put your hands behind your head.
3. Start twisting diagonally, touching your left knee with your right elbow.
4. Exhale as you twist and inhale as you lower your body to the mat (floor).
5. Then do this exercise while touching your right knee with your left elbow. To the other side.

Note: take your time and control every movement, try to feel every muscle with every repetition.

The benefits of the exercise: strengthens the rectus abdominis muscle, develops the internal muscles of the body, and also creates a load on the muscles of the upper body and arm muscles.

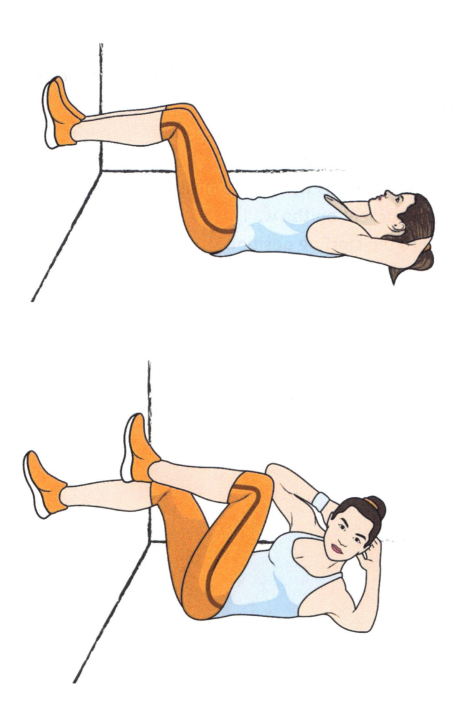

WALL PIKE CRUNCHES

How to do it:

1. Lie back on the mat with your buttocks fully against the wall (see illustration).
2. The legs are raised up, and pressed together.
3. Hands on the floor behind the head.
4. Try touching your ankles with your hands while keeping your arms straight and your feet on the wall.
5. Then return to the starting position.
6. Exhale as you rise and inhale as you lower yourself to the mat.

The benefits of the exercise: all abdominal and back muscles are trained and toned after doing this exercise.

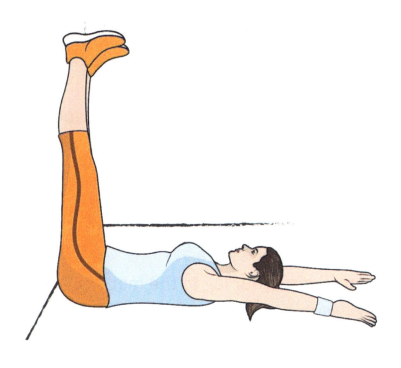
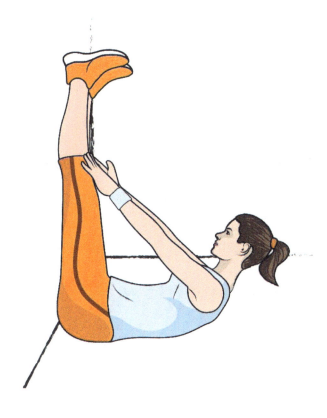

SUPERWOMAN

How to do it:

1. Lie on the mat facing the floor, legs straight, toes extended.
2. Place your left arm in front of you, bent at the elbow (see illustration).
3. Lean against the wall with your right hand.
4. As you exhale, lift your left leg up, pulling up with the tips of your toes without bending the knee.
5. While inhaling, lower your leg to the mat.
6. Then do this exercise with your *right leg* raised, and lean against the wall with your *left* hand.

Note: It is important to do this exercise slowly, inhaling deeply through the nose and exhaling through the mouth.

The benefits of the exercise: strengthening the muscles of the back, and buttocks, and improving posture.

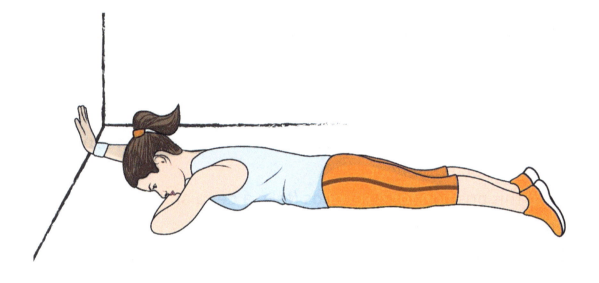

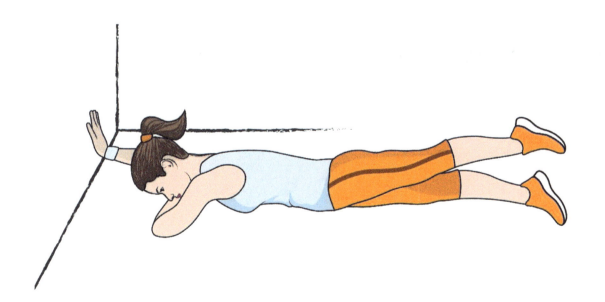

WALL TABLE TOP

How to do it:

1. Kneel on the mat, resting on your palms, arms straight.
2. Knees bent at a 90° angle, abdomen tightened, head straight.
3. Position yourself so that the wall is at a distance of an extended leg.
4. Inhale and as you exhale, straighten your right leg against the wall, touching it to maintain balance, while raising your left (opposite) arm parallel to the floor.
5. Hold this position for 4 seconds (take a deep and even breathe in and out of the air).
6. Lower your arm and leg to return to the starting position.
7. Then change the opposite leg and arm and hold it horizontally for 4 seconds.

The benefits of the exercise: toning of the torso and legs of the body.

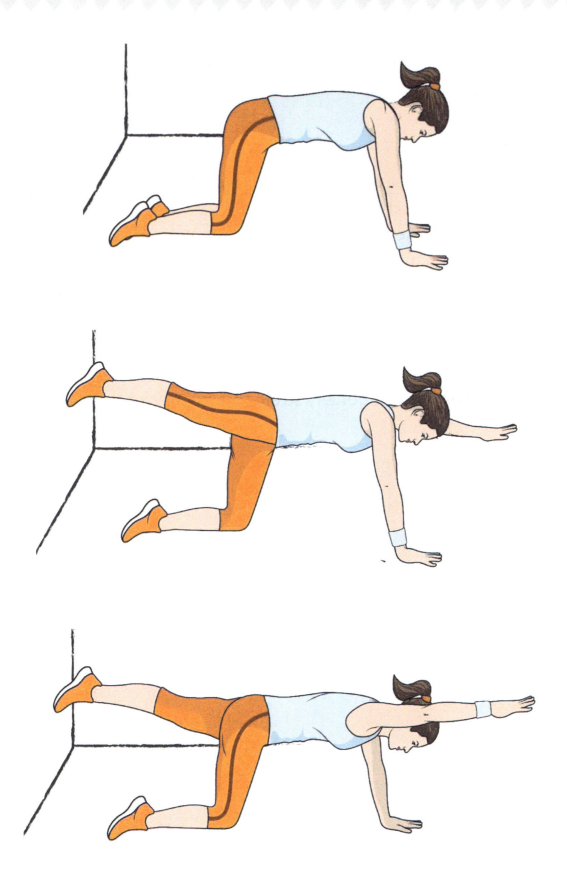

WALL SIDE LEG LIFT

How to do it:

1. Stand on the mat with your right knee and right hand on the mat or floor (see illustration).
2. Lean well against the wall with your left hand and extend your left leg parallel to the floor.
3. Start moving your leg up and down without touching the floor.
4. Repeat the same for the other leg.

Note: it is important to additionally strain the muscles of the buttocks and thighs.

The benefits of the exercise: this exercise is good for training the inner thigh.

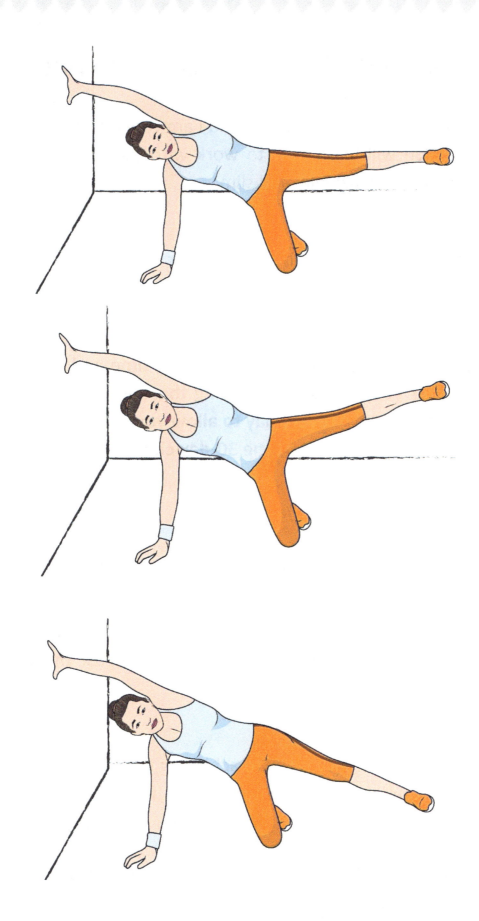

30-Day Body Sculpting Challenge

Today is your first day of training, and I am very glad that this book is in your hands. You will learn how to work with your body, feel it, and become more enduring, flexible, and slim.

Every day of training will bring you closer to the healthy and toned body you not only want but deserve.

Ideally, if you haven't exercised for a long time and feel tired and sore the day after your workout, try doing these exercises every other day for 5-10 days instead of every day to allow your body to adapt to the exercises. After that, you can start the 30-day challenge.

Notes:

Between each set of exercises, take a 30- to 50-second rest pause to ensure that you keep your heart rate high enough to make your workout effective for weight loss and cardio.

If you don't have an accessible wall for Pilates, you can *use the front door or a closet* (for standing exercises).

Keep in mind that consistency is key to achieving the best results. But, of course, listen to your body and give it more rest if it asks for it.

Shape your legs, abs and waist in these <u>30 days</u> and change your life forever!

DAY 1

EXERCISES	DURATION	PAGE
TILT THE BODY FORWARD	10 repetitions	14
WALL SINGLE LEG STRETCH (Left)	8 repetitions	20
WALL SINGLE LEG STRETCH (Right)	8 repetitions	22
SEATED TRUNK ROTATION	30 seconds	60
WALL PUSH-UP	8 repetitions	30
WALL CAT STRETCH	8 repetitions	44
WALL TABLE TOP	4 repetitions each side	68
WALL LEG RAISE + KICK BACK	6 repetitions each side	56

DAY 2

EXERCISES	DURATION	PAGE
WALL ANGELS	8 repetitions	58
LEGS-UP CRUNCH	6 repetitions	24
WALL BRIDGE	8 repetitions	16
SUPERWOMAN	4 repetitions each side	66
LIFTING ON THE TOES	8 repetitions	32
SMALL PELVIC LIFTS	10 repetitions	18
WALL TABLE TOP	4 repetitions each side	68
WALL LEG RAISE + KICK BACK	6 repetitions each side	56

DAY 3

EXERCISES	DURATION	PAGE
WALL LEG RAISE + KICK BACK	4 repetitions each side	56
WALL SINGLE LEG STRETCH (Left)	8 repetitions	20
WALL SINGLE LEG STRETCH (Right)	8 repetitions	22
FORWARD WALL SQUATS	8 repetitions	52
SEATED TRUNK ROTATION	8 repetitions	60
WALL SCISSOR	4 repetitions	38
WALL BICYCLE CRUNCHES	4 repetitions	62
WALL CAT STRETCH	4 repetitions	44
WALL CALF RAISES	10 repetitions	10

DAY 4

EXERCISES	DURATION	PAGE
TILT THE BODY FORWARD	10 repetitions	14
WALL BRIDGE	6 repetitions	16
WALL LEG LIFTS	8 repetitions	36
WALL SCISSOR	4 repetitions	38
WALL COBRA STRETCH	8 repetitions	26
SEATED TRUNK ROTATION	8 repetitions	60
WALL PUSH-UP	10 repetitions	30
LIFTING ON THE TOES	8 repetitions	32
WALL ANGELS	10 repetitions	58
SUPERWOMAN	4 repetitions each side	66

DAY 5

EXERCISES	DURATION	PAGE
WALL ANGELS	8 repetitions	58
WALL SINGLE LEG STRETCH (Left)	10 repetitions	20
WALL SINGLE LEG STRETCH (Right)	10 repetitions	22
SEATED TRUNK ROTATION	8 repetitions	60
WALL SQUATS ONE LEG	6 repetitions each side	34
WALL CALF RAISES	12 repetitions	10
WALL CAT STRETCH	8 repetitions	44
WALL BICYCLE CRUNCHES	6 repetitions each side	62
WALL SIDE LEG LIFT	4 repetitions each side	70
WALL SCISSOR	4 repetitions	38

DAY 6

EXERCISES	DURATION	PAGE
TILT THE BODY FORWARD	10 repetitions	14
WALL SQUATS	2 repetitions	40
WALL TABLE TOP	4 repetitions each side	68
WALL CAT STRETCH	8 repetitions	44
WALL BICYCLE CRUNCHES	4 repetitions each side	62
WALL PIKE CRUNCHES	10 repetitions	64
WALL CALF RAISES	10 repetitions	10
WALL ANGELS	8 repetitions	58
LEGS-UP CRUNCH	6 repetitions	24
WALL SCISSOR	4 repetitions	38

DAY 7

EXERCISES	DURATION	PAGE
WALL ANGELS	8 repetitions	58
LEGS-UP CRUNCH	6 repetitions	24
WALL SINGLE LEG STRETCH (Left)	8 repetitions	20
WALL SINGLE LEG STRETCH (Right)	8 repetitions	22
WALL BRIDGE	8 repetitions	16
WALL PLANK	2 repetitions	46
WALL PUSH-UP	8 repetitions	30
WALL CALF RAISES	16 repetitions	10
WALL SQUATS ONE LEG	6 repetitions each side	34
SEATED TRUNK ROTATION	8 repetitions	60

DAY 8

EXERCISES	DURATION	PAGE
WALL ANGELS	8 repetitions	58
WALL COBRA STRETCH	8 repetitions	26
WALL PIKE CRUNCHES	6 repetitions	64
WALL CALF RAISES	16 repetitions	10
WALL SINGLE LEG STRETCH (Left)	10 repetitions	20
WALL SINGLE LEG STRETCH (Right)	10 repetitions	22
WALL LEG LIFTS	10 repetitions	36

DAY 9

EXERCISES	DURATION	PAGE
TILT THE BODY FORWARD	10 repetitions	14
WALL BRIDGE	10 repetitions	16
WALL COBRA STRETCH	10 repetitions	26
SEATED TRUNK ROTATION	8 repetitions	60
WALL PUSH-UP	8 repetitions	30
WALL BICYCLE CRUNCHES	10 repetitions each side	62
WALL SCISSOR	4 repetitions	38
LEG LIFT WITH WALL SUPPORT	5 repetitions each side	50
WALL LEG RAISE + KICK BACK	8 repetitions each side	56
WALL ANGELS	8 repetitions	58

DAY 10

EXERCISES	DURATION	PAGE
WALL BRIDGE	6 repetitions	16
SMALL PELVIC LIFTS	6 repetitions	18
LEGS-UP CRUNCH	6 repetitions	24
SEATED TRUNK ROTATION	8 repetitions	60
ONE-LEGGED WALL SIT	2 repetitions each side	54
CLIMB A MOUNTAIN	2 repetitions	48
WALL SINGLE LEG STRETCH (Left)	8 repetitions	20
WALL SINGLE LEG STRETCH (Right)	8 repetitions	22
WALL SCISSOR	4 repetitions	38
WALL LEG LIFTS	10 repetitions	36
LEG LIFT WITH WALL SUPPORT	5 repetitions	50

DAY 11

EXERCISES	DURATION	PAGE
WALL PUSH-UP	8 repetitions	30
TILT THE BODY FORWARD	10 repetitions	14
WALL BRIDGE	8 repetitions	16
SMALL PELVIC LIFTS	6 repetitions	18
WALL SQUATS ONE LEG	6 repetitions each side	34
WALL LEG LIFTS	10 repetitions	36
SUPERWOMAN	6 repetitions each side	66
WALL TABLE TOP	4 repetitions each side	68
SEATED TRUNK ROTATION	8 repetitions	60
LIFTING ON THE TOES	8 repetitions	32
WALL CAT STRETCH	8 repetitions	44
WALL ANGELS	8 repetitions	58

DAY 12

EXERCISES	DURATION	PAGE
WALL BRIDGE	8 repetitions	16
WALL SINGLE LEG STRETCH (Left)	8 repetitions	20
WALL SINGLE LEG STRETCH (Right)	8 repetitions	22
WALL SIT HEEL RAISE	6 repetitions	42
WALL CAT STRETCH	8 repetitions	44
WALL TABLE TOP	4 repetitions each side	68
FORWARD WALL SQUATS	10 repetitions	52
WALL ANGELS	8 repetitions	58
WALL COBRA STRETCH	10 repetitions	26
TOE TOUCH CRUNCH	3 repetitions each side	28
LEG LIFT WITH WALL SUPPORT	5 repetitions each side	50
SUPERWOMAN	4 repetitions each side	66

DAY 13

EXERCISES	DURATION	PAGE
WALL LEG RAISE + KICK BACK	6 repetitions each side	56
WALL SINGLE LEG STRETCH (Left)	8 repetitions	20
WALL SINGLE LEG STRETCH (Right)	8 repetitions	22
WALL SQUATS ONE LEG	6 repetitions each side	34
SEATED TRUNK ROTATION	8 repetitions	60
WALL SCISSOR	6 repetitions	38
WALL SQUATS	2 repetitions	40
WALL CAT STRETCH	8 repetitions	44
LIFTING ON THE TOES	8 repetitions	32
WALL COBRA STRETCH	10 repetitions	26
WALL TABLE TOP	4 repetitions each side	68
LEG LIFT WITH WALL SUPPORT	5 repetitions each side	50
WALL ANGELS	8 repetitions	58

DAY 14

EXERCISES	DURATION	PAGE
TILT THE BODY FORWARD	10 repetitions	14
WALL BRIDGE	8 repetitions	16
SMALL PELVIC LIFTS	8 repetitions	18
WALL CAT STRETCH	8 repetitions	44
WALL SQUATS	2 repetitions	40
WALL SIT HEEL RAISE	6 repetitions	42
WALL LEG LIFTS	10 repetitions	36
WALL SCISSOR	6 repetitions	38
WALL PUSH-UP	8 repetitions	30
LIFTING ON THE TOES	8 repetitions	32
WALL SQUATS ONE LEG	4 repetitions each side	34
WALL LEG RAISE + KICK BACK	6 repetitions each side	56
WALL TABLE TOP	4 repetitions each side	68

DAY 15

EXERCISES	DURATION	PAGE
WALL ANGELS	8 repetitions	58
WALL PIKE CRUNCHES	6 repetitions	64
WALL BICYCLE CRUNCHES	4 repetitions each side	62
SEATED TRUNK ROTATION	8 repetitions	60
LEG LIFT WITH WALL SUPPORT	8 repetitions each side	50
TOE TOUCH CRUNCH	3 repetitions each side	28
WALL CAT STRETCH	10 repetitions	44
WALL PUSH-UP	8 repetitions	30
WALL LEG RAISE + KICK BACK	8 repetitions each side	56
FORWARD WALL SQUATS	8 repetitions	52
WALL SQUATS	2 repetitions	40
WALL SIT HEEL RAISE	6 repetitions	42

DAY 16

EXERCISES	DURATION	PAGE
WALL BRIDGE	12 repetitions	16
WALL PUSH-UP	10 repetitions	30
WALL LEG RAISE + KICK BACK	6 repetitions each side	56
WALL SQUATS	2 repetitions	40
WALL SIDE LEG LIFT	6 repetitions each side	70
FORWARD WALL SQUATS	10 repetitions	52

Perform 2-3 sets with a break of 30-50 seconds.

DAY 17

EXERCISES	DURATION	PAGE
WALL BICYCLE CRUNCHES	6 repetitions each side	62
LEG LIFT WITH WALL SUPPORT	5 repetitions each side	50
LEGS-UP CRUNCH	8 repetitions	24
SMALL PELVIC LIFTS	8 repetitions	18
WALL SCISSOR	4 repetitions	38

Perform 2-3 sets with a break of 30-50 seconds.

DAY 18

EXERCISES	DURATION	PAGE
WALL SINGLE LEG STRETCH (Left)	8 repetitions	20
WALL SINGLE LEG STRETCH (Right)	8 repetitions	22
WALL TABLE TOP	6 repetitions each side	68
WALL CAT STRETCH	10 repetitions	44
WALL PLANK	2 repetitions	46
WALL LEG LIFTS	10 repetitions	36
WALL LEG RAISE + KICK BACK	6 repetitions each side	56

Perform 2-3 sets with a break of 30-50 seconds.

DAY 19

EXERCISES	DURATION	PAGE
WALL PUSH-UP	10 repetitions	30
CLIMB A MOUNTAIN	2 repetitions	48
WALL BICYCLE CRUNCHES	6 repetitions each side	62
TOE TOUCH CRUNCH	4 repetitions each side	28
FORWARD WALL SQUATS	10 repetitions	52
WALL CALF RAISES	10 repetitions	10

Perform 2-3 sets with a break of 30-50 seconds.

DAY 20

EXERCISES	DURATION	PAGE
WALL LEG LIFTS	10 repetitions	36
TILT THE BODY FORWARD	10 repetitions	14
WALL SQUATS ONE LEG	6 repetitions each side	34
WALL PIKE CRUNCHES	6 repetitions	64
LIFTING ON THE TOES	8 repetitions	32

Perform 2-3 sets with a break of 30-50 seconds.

DAY 21

EXERCISES	DURATION	PAGE
WALL BRIDGE	12 repetitions	16
WALL SINGLE LEG STRETCH (Left)	10 repetitions	20
WALL SINGLE LEG STRETCH (Right)	10 repetitions	22
LEG LIFT WITH WALL SUPPORT	5 repetitions each side	50
WALL SQUATS	2 repetitions	40
WALL SIDE LEG LIFT	6 repetitions each side	70

Perform 2-3 sets with a break of 30-50 seconds.

DAY 22

EXERCISES	DURATION	PAGE
WALL SIT WITH LEG EXTENSION	6 repetitions	12
WALL PUSH-UP	10 repetitions	30
SUPERWOMAN	6 repetitions each side	66
WALL BRIDGE	8 repetitions	16
SMALL PELVIC LIFTS	6 repetitions	18
SEATED TRUNK ROTATION	8 repetitions	60

Perform 3-4 sets with a break of 30-50 seconds.

DAY 23

EXERCISES	DURATION	PAGE
WALL PIKE CRUNCHES	6 repetitions	64
FORWARD WALL SQUATS	10 repetitions	52
WALL ANGELS	8 repetitions	58
WALL LEG RAISE + KICK BACK	6 repetitions each side	56
WALL COBRA STRETCH	10 repetitions	26
WALL SQUATS ONE LEG	6 repetitions each side	34

Perform 3-4 sets with a break of 30-50 seconds.

DAY 24

EXERCISES	DURATION	PAGE
WALL BRIDGE	8 repetitions	16
TOE TOUCH CRUNCH	4 repetitions each side	28
WALL CAT STRETCH	10 repetitions	44
WALL PLANK	4 repetitions	46
WALL SINGLE LEG STRETCH (Left)	10 repetitions	20
WALL SINGLE LEG STRETCH (Right)	10 repetitions	22
WALL SIDE LEG LIFT	6 repetitions each side	70

Perform 3-4 sets with a break of 30-50 seconds.

DAY 25

EXERCISES	DURATION	PAGE
FORWARD WALL SQUATS	10 repetitions	52
WALL PUSH-UP	10 repetitions	30
ONE-LEGGED WALL SIT	2 repetitions each side	54
WALL PIKE CRUNCHES	8 repetitions	64
WALL SCISSOR	4 repetitions	38

Perform 3-4 sets with a break of 30-50 seconds.

DAY 26

EXERCISES	DURATION	PAGE
WALL SQUATS	2 repetitions	40
WALL LEG LIFTS	10 repetitions	36
LIFTING ON THE TOES	8 repetitions	32
WALL BICYCLE CRUNCHES	6 repetitions each side	62
WALL SIT WITH LEG EXTENSION	6 repetitions	12

Perform 3-4 sets with a break of 30-50 seconds.

DAY 27

EXERCISES	DURATION	PAGE
WALL ANGELS	8 repetitions	58
LEG LIFT WITH WALL SUPPORT	5 repetitions each side	50
WALL SIT HEEL RAISE	6 repetitions	42
WALL COBRA STRETCH	10 repetitions	26
WALL TABLE TOP	6 repetitions each side	68
WALL CALF RAISES	10 repetitions	10

Perform 3-4 sets with a break of 30-50 seconds.

DAY 28

EXERCISES	DURATION	PAGE
TILT THE BODY FORWARD	10 repetitions	14
WALL SINGLE LEG STRETCH (Left)	10 repetitions	20
WALL SINGLE LEG STRETCH (Right)	10 repetitions	22
FORWARD WALL SQUATS	10 repetitions	52
WALL PUSH-UP	10 repetitions	30
LEGS-UP CRUNCH	8 repetitions	24

Perform 3-4 sets with a break of 30-50 seconds.

DAY 29

EXERCISES	DURATION	PAGE
WALL LEG RAISE + KICK BACK	6 repetitions each side	56
SEATED TRUNK ROTATION	8 repetitions	60
WALL SQUATS ONE LEG	6 repetitions each side	34
WALL COBRA STRETCH	10 repetitions	26
TOE TOUCH CRUNCH	4 repetitions each side	28
WALL CAT STRETCH	10 repetitions	44

Perform 3-4 sets with a break of 30-50 seconds.

DAY 30

EXERCISES	DURATION	PAGE
WALL BRIDGE	8 repetitions	16
WALL PUSH-UP	10 repetitions	30
WALL CAT STRETCH	10 repetitions	44
WALL PLANK	4 repetitions	46
WALL SINGLE LEG STRETCH (Left)	10 repetitions	20
WALL SINGLE LEG STRETCH (Right)	10 repetitions	22

Perform 3-4 sets with a break of 30-50 seconds.

Tracking the 30-day challenge

Consistency is the key to success.

Day	Training done ✓	Energy level (high, medium, low)	Mood (good, normal, tired)
1			
2			
3			
4			
5			
6			
7			
8			
9			
10			
11			
12			
13			
14			
15			
16			
17			
18			
19			
20			
21			
22			
23			
24			
25			

26			
27			
28			
29			
30			

PDF BONUS:

Get your PDF bonus with all the exercises and instructions + 4 additional workout programs. PDF works great on your computer or phone.

Just send me a confirmation of your book purchase by email:

goreadandmakeit@gmail.com

Made in the USA
Coppell, TX
08 October 2023

22550564R00059